A Complete Guide to Acupuncture Points

The Practical Guide to Heal Yourself of Every Common Illnesses Using the Therapeutic Needle Sticks

Dani Twain

Contents

CHAPTER 11: Faq: Common Queries Regarding Acupuncture

Introduction

Acupuncture is rooted in an understanding of the intricate network of energy channels, known as meridians, that course through the human body, facilitating the flow of vital energy. These meridians are intimately linked with internal organs, and any imbalance of energy within them can disrupt bodily functions. Acupuncturists possess the ability to regulate this energy flow by stimulating specific points along these meridians.

Each acupuncture point comprises a region of the skin and underlying subcutaneous tissue, characterized by a complex arrangement of microstructures such as blood vessels, nerves, and connective tissue cells. These structures create an active zone capable of influencing nerve endings and facilitating communication between the skin and internal organs.

Distinctive features of acupuncture points include heightened oxygen absorption, elevated temperature, and reduced electrical resistance compared to surrounding skin areas. The size of these points varies depending on the individual's state, with diameters typically around one centimeter in waking individuals, slightly smaller in sleep, and potentially larger during periods of psycho-emotional stress or acute somatic illnesses.

Precise manipulation of acupuncture points can yield therapeutic benefits, ranging from pain relief and migraine management to addressing issues such as knee pain, neck pain, back pain, weight loss, depression, birth preparation, allergies, neurodermatitis, smoking cessation, Parkinson's disease, sleep disorders, stress-related complaints, and tinnitus. Additionally, acupuncture has found application in modern medicine for treating a broad spectrum of neurological, somatic, and psychosomatic disorders, contributing to overall health and well-being.

Chapter 1

Understanding Acupuncture

Acupuncture stands as a well-established therapeutic technique, employing the insertion of fine needles, each no thicker than a strand of hair, into specific points on the body to address various medical conditions. Originating approximately 5,000 years ago in the Sino-Uyghur region, its foundational principles and application methods have endured over time. In our contemporary context, its practice is restricted to licensed medical professionals sanctioned by the Ministry of Health. While potential side effects such as localized infections or fluctuations in blood pressure may arise, these risks are mitigated under the skilled hands of qualified practitioners.

One of acupuncture's notable attributes is its minimal risk of adverse effects, coupled with diagnostic approaches that encourage patient engagement and a recognition that ailments affect the entire body, fostering a holistic treatment approach. Thus, acupuncture serves as a potent therapeutic tool in our arsenal, particularly in addressing various forms of pain and other medical conditions that afflict our patients.

Chapter 2

The Origin of Acupuncture

The origins of acupuncture trace back to ancient Chinese medical texts dating as far back as the 3rd century BC. One such text, the "Huang Di Nei Jing" from 221 BC, documented 295 specific points on the human body believed to possess therapeutic properties when needles were inserted into them, aiding in the treatment of various ailments.

Initially focused on alleviating pain, acupuncture gradually evolved to address more intricate medical conditions. By the middle of the 3rd century AD, the treatise "Jia and Jing" expanded the repertoire to include descriptions of 649 acupuncture points.

The philosophical underpinnings of Taoism significantly influenced the development of acupuncture. Taoist concepts concerning the flow of vital energy within the body and its alignment with the natural rhythms of the universe shaped the understanding of bioactive points as gateways to the body's energy system, capable of harmonizing the balance between Yin and Yang energies.

Initially fashioned from materials like stone, bamboo, or bone, acupuncture needles evolved over time to primarily comprise metal.

As medical practitioners delved deeper into the practice, they observed that stimulating different points on the body could affect the functioning of specific organs, leading to the systematization of knowledge. This categorization resulted in the identification of meridians, lines connecting points associated with particular organs.

Aligned with Taoist philosophy, it was postulated that vital energy flowed along these meridians, nurturing the body's organs. Moreover, additional meridians were discovered, serving as reservoirs for energy accumulation. Among these, two primary meridians, known as the main channels, were deemed responsible for maintaining the overall equilibrium of Yin and Yang energies within the body.

Acupuncture in China

The evolution of acupuncture took dual pathways. Firstly, practitioners continually unearthed novel bioactive points, documented in atlases. Secondly, they innovated diverse treatment protocols and needle techniques, yielding increasingly varied therapeutic outcomes. It became evident that organ function could be modulated not only via its own meridian but also through those of other organs, theoretically represented by the Five Primary Elements pentagram.

Initially, knowledge transmission occurred from mentor to disciple, fostering diverse traditions. However, in 1076, these traditions coalesced into a unified school. By this time, Chinese practitioners had identified 657 bioactive points, leading to standardization of acupuncture methods and techniques.

Acupuncture in Tibetan and Mongolian Medicine

In Tibetan medicine, needle therapy initially played a subordinate role and was primarily utilized when herbal remedies yielded unsatisfactory results. The assimilation of Chinese treatment methods into Tibetan medicine likely transpired during the 8th-9th centuries, coinciding with Tibet's expansion into Chinese territories.

Subsequently, in the 12th century, Genghis Khan's conquest of Tibet facilitated the dissemination of Tibetan medicine into Mongolia. The descendants of Genghis Khan further expanded their dominion into China, indirectly fostering the amalgamation of Tibetan herbal medicine and Chinese acupuncture, thereby giving rise to Mongolian medicine.

However, acupuncture did not experience significant advancement within Tibetan medicine. Preferring acupressure and moxibustion, Tibetan practitioners, while embracing the theory of body meridians and bioactive points from Chinese medicine, opted for alternative modalities of influence.

In the 1950s, acupuncture made significant inroads into Western countries, where practitioners encountered a distinct array of ailments and underlying causes compared to their Eastern counterparts. This necessitated adaptations and innovations in acupuncture techniques, sparking its evolution.

For instance, conditions like osteochondrosis, uncommon in Eastern regions and typically associated with advanced age, became prevalent in the West, often manifesting in middle age. Addressing such shifts demanded the formulation of novel acupuncture protocols tailored to Western health challenges.

Moreover, acupuncture gained scientific validation in Western contexts, with research confirming its impact on cerebral cortex regions, interneuronal networks, immune responses, and neurohormonal balance. This scientific grounding facilitated its integration into evidence-based medical practices.

Chapter 3

Types of Acupuncture

Contemporary acupuncture encompasses various approaches, not all of which adhere strictly to traditional acupuncture principles. The choice of technique depends on the stage of pathological conditions, with different methods offering varying degrees of intensity in point stimulation. Alongside traditional acupuncture, modern practices include:

1. Acupressure and Shiatsu massage involve finger and palm pressure.

2. Su-jok focuses on needle therapy applied solely to the hands and feet.

3. Vacuum therapy employs cupping massage techniques.

4. Laser therapy targets acupuncture points with a laser beam.

5. Electropuncture utilizes electrodes to deliver electric currents to the points.

6. Baunsheitism entails the simultaneous insertion of multiple needles, followed by surface treatment with skin-irritating substances.

7. Moxibustion involves warming inserted needles.

Moreover, unconventional methods incorporate living organisms for therapeutic purposes. For instance, hirudotherapy employs leeches to stimulate biologically active points, while apitherapy uses bee stings. This diverse array of options enables practitioners to tailor treatments to individual needs, optimizing therapeutic outcomes.

Chapter 4

Mechanisms of Acupuncture

While we recognize the efficacy of acupuncture, fully grasping its underlying mechanisms remains a challenge. Attempting to understand acupuncture's mode of action through the lens of observable science, rooted in Newtonian principles, poses a significant hurdle. Acupuncture posits the existence of an imperceptible energy balance within the body, attributing most ailments to disruptions in this equilibrium. By restoring this disrupted balance, relief from illness is purportedly achieved. Advancements in Quantum Physics may offer insights that bolster our comprehension of acupuncture's mechanism of action.

Nevertheless, numerous studies supported by modern medicine and science suggest that acupuncture influences the nervous system, leading to the release of endorphins and other biochemicals. It has been observed to stimulate the secretion of endogenous pain-relieving substances, modulate hormone levels positively, enhance local blood circulation, bolster the immune system, and induce muscle relaxation. In essence, acupuncture appears to harness the body's innate healing mechanisms at the bioelectrical level.

Chapter 5

Application of Acupuncture

Following a thorough examination, specific combinations of acupuncture points are chosen based on the diagnosed condition or ailment. Sterile needles, typically measuring between 1 to 4 centimeters, are then inserted into these selected points. These needles are left in place for approximately 20 to 60 minutes. The key consideration lies in the careful selection of points and the precise application technique employed. Various methods such as laser therapy, electroacupuncture, and moxibustion may complement needle insertion. While some discomfort may be experienced upon needle insertion, most patients report minimal to no pain during the session.

Chapter 6

Applications of Acupuncture in Treating Various Conditions

In clinical settings, acupuncture is frequently employed to alleviate pain, with its efficacy extending to over 100 different conditions. While it enjoys popularity in aiding weight loss and smoking cessation, its primary application lies in pain relief. Commonly treated ailments include lower back pain, neck pain, and unilateral headaches. These areas constitute the primary focus of acupuncture therapy within our clinic.

Additionally, acupuncture proves beneficial in addressing a spectrum of conditions ranging from anxiety, stress, and self-doubt to facial paralysis, sleep disorders, and digestive issues like irritable bowel syndrome and fibromyalgia. Its therapeutic utility extends to restless leg syndrome as well. The underlying philosophy of acupuncture attributes these disturbances to disruptions in the body's energy circulation within its channels, which are invisible to the naked eye. Acupuncture treatment seeks to regulate the flow within these channels, restoring balance and promoting healing.

Chapter 7

Contrasting Acupuncture and Acupressure

Acupuncture, a well-known practice, involves the insertion of specialized needles into specific points on the body. This alternative healing method, rooted in traditional Chinese medicine (TCM), is typically administered by trained specialists. In Germany, practitioners from various medical disciplines, as well as alternative therapists, undergo additional training to qualify for acupuncture practice.

It's worth noting that alongside traditional acupuncture, there are now self-acupuncture devices available, such as acupuncture pens. These tools provide individuals with the means to perform acupuncture on themselves, offering an alternative to traditional needle insertion.

In contrast, acupressure does not involve the use of needles. Instead, practitioners apply pressure to acupuncture points using their fingers.

Acupressure is deeply ingrained in Chinese culture, with many individuals possessing basic knowledge of this therapeutic technique. While Western medicine often relies on pharmaceuticals for pain relief, acupressure leverages targeted finger pressure to alleviate discomfort and promote wellness.

Chapter 8

Advantages of Acupuncture

Acupuncture in Pregnancy:

Acupuncture emerges as a beneficial approach for alleviating discomfort during pregnancy. Particularly, it aids in mitigating the common nausea experienced within the initial trimester, while also addressing circulatory issues and sleep disturbances. Furthermore, acupuncture plays a role in preparing the perineum for childbirth and facilitating cervical dilation.

Acupuncture for Pain Management and Migraines:

This therapeutic modality demonstrates notable efficacy in addressing conditions such as tendonitis, migraines, osteoarthritis, and arthritis.

Acupuncture for Treating Functional Disorders:

Acupuncture presents promise in managing functional disorders, including allergies, hypertension, dermatological conditions, digestive ailments, among others.

Chapter 9

Acupuncture: Scientifically Validated and Endorsed by the WHO

In contemporary times, traditional Chinese medicine, including acupuncture, holds a significant position in the roster of traditional healing modalities recognized by the World Health Organization (WHO). The efficacy of acupuncture has undergone rigorous scientific scrutiny and has been increasingly integrated into medical practices across Europe over the past few decades.

Acupuncture has notably entrenched itself as a targeted complementary therapy alongside conventional medicine, spanning various domains of alternative healing modalities.

Furthermore, numerous scientific investigations have corroborated the effectiveness of acupuncture, unveiling intriguing correlations. Anatomical investigations reveal that the majority of acupuncture points precisely align with nerve emergence points within muscle tissue. Stimulating these points triggers the release of hormones and activates pain-inhibitory mechanisms within the brain and spinal cord via neurotransmitters.

Precise stimulation of acupuncture points can modulate the functions of organs, muscles, skin, and tendons. Techniques such as slight rotation, lifting, lowering, stroking, or rocking of acupuncture needles can augment the therapeutic effects of acupuncture.

Chapter **10**

Acupuncture for Specific Conditions

Addressing Hay Fever through Acupuncture

Acupuncture has emerged as a complementary therapy for hay fever, aiming to alleviate symptoms by addressing the blockage of life energy in the upper respiratory organs, as per traditional Chinese medicine principles.

Promising Results in Hay Fever Management with Acupuncture

A study conducted at the Berlin Charite involving approximately 5,000 hay fever patients showcased encouraging outcomes. Around 80 percent of participants experienced significant symptom improvement, accompanied by a notable enhancement in their overall quality of life.

Understanding Hay Fever from an Energetic Perspective

In the realm of Traditional Chinese Medicine (TCM), hay fever is attributed to a weakness in Wei Qi, which denotes a deficiency in the body's defense mechanisms. This deficiency can stem from congenital factors or develop over time due to various influences.

Furthermore, inadequate treatment of wind-cold exposure along the lung meridian can lead to the accumulation of lung energy (lung Qi), impeding the free flow of Qi in the upper respiratory tract. Additionally, dysfunction in the earth element (involving the stomach, spleen, and pancreas) contributes to heightened moisture production, excessive secretions, and irritations such as eye and nasal mucosa redness and itching.

Dietary Considerations in Managing Hay Fever

According to TCM principles, dietary choices play a crucial role in managing hay fever symptoms. Foods believed to exacerbate symptoms include:

- Iced drinks and cold foods
- Cold beverages during meals
- Cold muesli with milk
- Excessive consumption of raw foods and fruits

- Heavy meat-based meals in the evening

- Sugary treats, cakes, ice cream, and chocolate

- Sour and cold foods

- Dairy products like sour milk, cheese, and milk

- Tomatoes, cucumbers, legume sprouts, and tropical fruits

- Processed foods, ready-made sauces, canned goods, and low-calorie products

- Frozen meals, microwave dinners

- Artificial sweeteners and margarine

- Highly processed cooking oils

- Excessive bread consumption

- Sausages and processed meats

- Fruit juices, wheat beer, lemonade, and cola

- Pork

- Refined flour products such as white bread, rolls, pizza dough, and pasta.

Acupuncture for Hay Fever

Acupuncture aims to strengthen weakened organ systems and restore balance to lung energy, thereby addressing factors contributing to hay fever such as heat, humidity, or wind. Specific acupuncture points, like Ma 40, are targeted to dissolve mucus stagnation and reduce excessive mucus production.

Treatment Process

Hay fever typically requires 10-12 acupuncture sessions, ideally initiated 4-6 weeks before the anticipated onset of symptoms. In cases of severe symptoms, sessions may be scheduled twice weekly initially, with a transition to once weekly after approximately 4 weeks.

In the first year of treatment, a reduction of symptoms by around 50% is commonly observed. By the second year, many individuals may experience complete relief from symptoms.

Acupuncture for Anxiety and Fear

Acupuncture offers notable effectiveness in alleviating anxiety, targeting both its mental and physical manifestations. Anxiety is a common human experience, triggered by significant life events such as meetings, exams, or negotiations. Acupuncture can help soothe nerves and alleviate the chest's tightness often associated with anxiety.

However, in the context of addressing chronic anxiety and fear, acupuncture plays a crucial role in improving overall quality of life. Various conditions and ailments can induce persistent feelings of fear, sometimes escalating into debilitating panic attacks if left untreated.

In severe cases, individuals may experience sudden and unexplained panic episodes, intrusive thoughts, nightmares, and physical distress.

Fortunately, there exist diverse therapeutic modalities to aid individuals with anxiety, among which acupuncture stands out. Before delving deeper into the efficacy of acupuncture in anxiety reduction, it's important to recognize the five primary types of anxiety:

1. Panic Disorder: Characterized by intense, sudden episodes of fear, accompanied by physical symptoms like palpitations, chest pain, shortness of breath, dizziness, abdominal discomfort, and a sense of impending doom. In Chinese medicine, this condition is often associated with heart-heat-blood syndrome.

2. Obsessive-Compulsive Disorder (OCD): Involves persistent, uncontrollable obsessions, compulsions, or behaviors. In Chinese

medicine, OCD is linked to Spleen Yin deficiency, where the imbalance in Yin Spleen manifests as obsessive thoughts and actions.

Acupuncture for reducing anxiety and fear typically entails strengthening Spleen Yin to restore balance.

Reaction to Severe Stress and Adjustment Disorders

Symptoms resembling panic attacks, such as nightmares, intrusive memories, emotional numbness, depression, and feelings of anger and irritability, often manifest in individuals who have experienced trauma or violence, including witnesses to such events. In some cases, individuals may not have been directly involved but have a family member affected. From the perspective of Traditional Chinese Medicine (TCM), this condition signifies an imbalance in energy flow. Acupuncture aids in restoring the harmonious flow of energy.

Phobias

There are two main types of phobias. Social phobia involves an irrational fear of public judgment or rejection, leading to social avoidance and isolation. Specific phobia, such as arachnophobia (fear of spiders), represents a fear of particular objects or situations. In TCM, these fears are attributed to Heart Yin deficiency.

Generalized Anxiety

Generalized anxiety manifests as a pervasive sense of unease unrelated to external factors. Symptoms may include constant nervousness, tremors, headaches, muscle tension, sweating, palpitations, dizziness, and chest discomfort. Patients often fear serious illness, potentially progressing through various TCM syndromes, such as Yin deficiency in the early stages, evolving into Spleen or Heart Yin deficiency.

The distinguishing aspect of Traditional Chinese Medicine and acupuncture lies in the personalized diagnosis of an individual's syndrome, informing a tailored treatment plan. Unlike medication, which primarily addresses symptoms, acupuncture for anxiety and worry targets the underlying disharmony causing the anxiety.

Acupuncture for Arthritis: Effectiveness and Procedure

The effectiveness of acupuncture for arthritis varies based on several factors, including the patient's unique condition, the type and stage of arthritis, and the expertise of the acupuncturist. While some individuals may experience immediate relief after a single session, others may require multiple treatments for noticeable improvement.

Benefits of acupuncture for arthritis may include:

- Pain relief and inflammation reduction
- Enhancement of overall physical and emotional well-being

However, it's important to note that the effects of acupuncture may be temporary, necessitating regular sessions over time to achieve sustained results. As one of several treatment options for arthritis, its efficacy varies among individuals.

Before undergoing acupuncture for arthritis, it's advisable to consult with a healthcare professional, preferably an Alternative Medical Center physician, who can provide a thorough assessment and recommend the most suitable approach based on your specific condition and medical history.

Procedure of Acupuncture for Arthritis:

1. Assessment: The practitioner evaluates the patient's condition, considering their medical background, arthritis symptoms, and other relevant factors to determine the optimal acupuncture approach.

2. Patient Preparation: The patient assumes a comfortable position,

typically lying down or sitting, depending on the targeted body area. They may also receive information about the procedure and its expected outcomes.

3. Needle Insertion: Thin needles are delicately inserted into specific points on the body, either near the site of pain or other acupuncture points associated with arthritis symptoms. These needles may remain in place for several minutes to half an hour or longer, as determined by the practitioner's approach.

4. Needle Manipulation: In some instances, the acupuncturist may manipulate the needles by rotating, oscillating, or gently lifting them to enhance stimulation.

5. Needle Removal: Upon completion of the procedure, the needles are carefully removed from the patient's body.

6. Rest and Observation: Following the treatment, the patient rests for a designated period while the practitioner observes their response to the acupuncture session.

Acupuncture for Back Pain

Acupuncture emerges as a promising treatment for various types of pain, including back pain, limb pain, facial pain, and headaches. Its efficacy in addressing such conditions has been recognized for centuries.

In the late 20th century, acupuncture gained significant attention in Europe, the USA, and Canada, particularly for alleviating back pain. This interest stems partly from concerns over contraindications and potential complications associated with synthetic medications.

The process of acupuncture treatment for back pain involves precisely inserting sterile acupuncture needles into specific active zones responsible for various bodily functions. These zones typically contain nerve fibers, nerve endings, or clusters of specialized receptors, often with reflex responses linked to internal organs. In certain cases, needles may target trigger points, areas of localized muscle contraction or inflammation. Notably, researchers such as Travel and Simons made notable contributions to understanding pain reflexes in the body, with Travel notably serving as John F. Kennedy's personal physician, addressing the President's chronic back pain.

The therapeutic mechanism of acupuncture operates through the generation of impulses upon needle insertion, eliciting secondary reflex reactions. Depending on the practitioner's technique, these reactions can modulate muscle tone, enhance blood circulation, and improve tissue nutrition, primarily benefiting the autonomic nervous system.

Acupuncture stands as a potent non-pharmacological intervention for pain management, extending even to spinal and back pain. In China, acupuncture has been employed to facilitate surgical procedures, achieving complete anesthesia for limb and internal organ surgeries.

Acupuncture can yield several benefits, including:

- Pain relief
- Enhanced tissue and cerebral blood flow
- Regulation of blood pressure
- Reduction of muscle tension during painful muscle contractions

In certain cases, the efficacy of acupuncture rivals that of conventional medications like analgesics, muscle relaxants (e.g., mydocalm, sirdalud), and vascular drugs.

Addressing Coughs (Both Wet and Dry) with Acupuncture

Efficiently managing both wet and dry coughs can be achieved through acupuncture, Chinese medicine, and the use of essential oils. As a Chinese medicine practitioner based in Lyon, I demonstrate how straightforward interventions can effectively address these types of coughs. Employing a combination of techniques, including acupuncture and massage with essential oils and floral waters, proves beneficial in combating coughs, whether oily or dry.

Amidst concerns like flu, colds, and other winter-related ailments, a holistic approach integrating acupuncture-tuina and aromatherapy becomes essential.

Flu and colds represent viral infections affecting the upper respiratory tract. Within Traditional Chinese Medicine (TCM), these conditions are attributed to an external wind invasion, which may manifest as wind-heat, wind-cold, wind-heat-humidity, or wind-heat-dryness, with wind-cold and wind-heat being the most common. Symptoms typically include fever (or chills), runny nose, fatigue, sweating, rhinitis, colds, headache, and wet or dry cough.

In Chinese medicine, the Lung meridian, along with the Large Intestine meridian coupled to it, is particularly susceptible to such invasions. Additionally, the Spleen and Stomach meridians are sensitive to wind attacks.

Acupuncture-tuina, involving therapeutic massage of acupuncture points tailored by the acupuncturist's expertise, proves effective in alleviating flu or cold symptoms, such as headaches and general discomfort (fever, fatigue, cough, body aches).

Numerous acupuncture points in Chinese medicine actively target flu-related issues. Examples include GI4 (Large Intestine), GI11, V13 (Bladder), V12, P7 (Lung), P11, and E36 (Stomach).

In addition, incorporating essential oils (aromatherapy) applied to acupuncture points and appropriate massage areas (via tuina) enhances well-being and therapeutic efficacy. Essential oils play a significant role in alleviating flu symptoms, with some scientific authors like Faucon, Franchomme, and Baudoux even likening them to plant antibiotics.

Tailoring to individual constitutions and backgrounds, a selection of essential oils can be diluted in organic vegetable oil. Options include Ravintsara (Cinnamomun camphora), Noble laurel (Laurus nobilis), Tea tree (Melaleuca alternifolia), and Radiated eucalyptus (Eucalyptus radiata).

Caution is advised, as certain individuals may have allergies to specific essential oils or encounter contraindications (e.g., children, pregnant or breastfeeding women, and various pathologies). The choice of oils is determined through collaborative discussions.

Furthermore, I recommend olfactotherapy (smell therapy) during sessions. The potent scents of Scots pine (Pinus sylvestrie) and peppermint (Mentha piperita) facilitate nasal decongestion and alleviate persistent headaches. A few drops of these oils on a tissue for inhalation can often provide relief from flu symptoms.

Acupuncture and the aspiration for parenthood: Holistic assistance for hopeful parents

For numerous couples, the dream of having a child represents a significant life goal. However, the journey toward realizing this dream is often more complex than anticipated. When faced with the disappointment of unfulfilled parenthood, couples commonly experience profound frustration and emotional strain. In such challenging times, many turn to additional sources of support, and acupuncture emerges as a valuable ally.

Acupuncture and the desire for parenthood: Mechanisms of action

According to traditional Chinese medicine, the inability to conceive is viewed as a bodily imbalance. Acupuncture endeavors to rectify this imbalance by enhancing blood circulation, regulating hormone levels, and mitigating stress—all of which can impact the process of conception.

Enhancement of blood flow: Optimal blood circulation in the reproductive organs is pivotal for successful conception. Acupuncture interventions can bolster blood flow to these areas, potentially enhancing the quality of both eggs and sperm.

Regulation of hormones: Hormonal irregularities can detrimentally affect fertility. Acupuncture offers a means to harmonize hormones such as FSH (follicle-stimulating hormone) and LH (luteinizing hormone), pivotal for ovulation and egg maturation.

Stress alleviation: Stress exerts a negative influence on fertility. Acupuncture endeavors to alleviate stress and promote overall well-being, fostering a conducive environment for conception.

Timing of acupuncture sessions for aspiring parents

Optimal outcomes are often realized when individuals commence acupuncture prior to actively attempting to conceive. It is advisable to initiate sessions at least three months before embarking on conception efforts. This timeframe allows the body ample opportunity to respond to treatment and prepare for the journey of pregnancy.

Acupuncture: Safe and natural assistance for prospective parents

Acupuncture represents a safe and natural avenue for bolstering the desire for parenthood. It can facilitate the body's readiness for conception, alleviate stress, and rectify hormonal imbalances. Countless couples have recounted positive experiences with acupuncture, citing enhanced fertility and the eventual realization of their parenthood aspirations.

Acupuncture for Migraines and Headaches

Many individuals attest to the therapeutic efficacy of acupuncture in averting migraine attacks. Indeed, scientific research indicates that the frequency of migraines often diminishes in the initial period following acupuncture therapy. However, sham acupuncture (sometimes referred to as a placebo treatment) yields similar effectiveness. Put simply:

Scientific evidence supports the beneficial role of acupuncture in preventing episodic migraines.

This positive outcome is observed even when migraine patients undergo sham acupuncture, rather than traditional Chinese acupuncture.

The extent to which acupuncture aids in chronic migraines remains inadequately investigated from a scientific standpoint.

Furthermore, there is indication that acupuncture is effective primarily for individuals who possess a fundamentally optimistic outlook toward it. Nonetheless, this should not deter those considering treatment.

Acupuncture Points for Migraines

The selection of acupuncture points for treating migraines varies based on individual circumstances. Ideally, the therapist obtains a comprehensive understanding of the ailment, identifying any blockages in the patient's energy pathways, and subsequently places needles at various points accordingly. For instance, the bile or liver ducts are commonly implicated.

In the accompanying illustration, locations for needle insertion for migraines are depicted—always on both sides of the body as acupuncture points are symmetrical. Traditional Chinese Medicine (TCM) delineates functional circuits associated with different organs, traversing specific parts or the entirety of the body. The acupuncture points stimulated in migraine cases are situated along these energy pathways.

Legend:

GB = Gallbladder functional circuit

LU = Lung functional circuit

LE = Liver functional area

The numerical annotations correspond to individual acupuncture points within the respective functional area.

The objective of needle stimulation is to restore the body to a state of harmony—referred to by Chinese scholars as the inner balance of Yin and Yang. Congested energy is encouraged to flow anew, rectifying imbalances between excesses and deficiencies.

Crucially, during needle application, minimal interference is ensured to enable patients to fully relax, with many even drifting off to sleep.

Our Recommendation

Consider giving acupuncture a try to determine its effectiveness for you. However, if you notice no improvement after several sessions, consider exploring alternative prophylactic methods such as biofeedback therapy or progressive muscle relaxation.

Acupuncture for Other Headaches

In addition to migraines, acupuncture can also be beneficial for tension headaches stemming from factors like poor posture or stress. However, acupuncture does not seem to impact cluster headaches positively. In fact, it might even trigger an attack.

Pros and Cons of Acupuncture Compared to Medication

Acupuncture can serve as an effective means to prevent migraines, offering the advantage of avoiding concerns about side effects. If acupuncture doesn't yield results, you can easily explore other options. However, its drawback lies in its inconsistency, as it doesn't work for every individual. Some experts question its efficacy, suggesting that participants' preconceived beliefs might skew evaluation. Another limitation of acupuncture is its inability to provide immediate relief during acute migraine attacks.

In contrast, drug prophylaxis carries the risk of adverse effects due to prolonged medication usage and may not be effective for everyone. In such cases, acupuncture presents itself as a viable alternative.

Cost and Duration of Acupuncture for Migraines and Other Headaches
Acupuncture for migraines or tension-related headaches typically isn't covered by statutory health insurance. Patients with migraines typically bear

the costs, ranging from 30 to 70 euros per session. Treatment frequency usually involves two sessions per week lasting 20 to 30 minutes each. Initial improvements are often observed after approximately seven to eight sessions, with a complete treatment spanning around 15 sessions.

Post-Acupuncture Treatment Considerations

If minimal improvement is observed after one treatment cycle, another cycle can be pursued. Successful acupuncture therapy often involves periodic maintenance sessions every few months. If migraines or headaches resurface after months or years, prompt acupuncture repetition is advised.

Acupuncture for Managing Hot Flashes

Acupuncture stands out as a remarkably effective alternative therapy for alleviating menopausal symptoms, particularly hot flashes. This non-invasive technique not only prevents excessive reactions within the body but also releases energy blockages, fostering a harmonious flow of energy throughout the entire system. In many instances, acupuncture demonstrates exceptional efficacy in mitigating hot flashes, offering relief that is both potent and devoid of adverse effects.

Among naturopathic modalities, acupuncture ranks high in addressing menopausal symptoms like hot flashes. In fact, research conducted at Henry Ford Hospital in Detroit and presented at a meeting of the American Society for Therapeutic Radiology and Oncology underscores acupuncture's superiority over conventional drug therapy in this regard.

Acupuncture for Hot Flashes During Breast Cancer Treatment with Tamoxifen

Notably, acupuncture has emerged as a preferable option compared to medication, especially for managing hot flashes induced by breast cancer treatment, particularly the use of tamoxifen. Tamoxifen, by reducing estrogen effects, induces menopausal symptoms like hot flashes in breast cancer patients, rendering conventional hormone replacement therapy impractical.

While antidepressants are sometimes prescribed to alleviate menopausal symptoms, they may introduce undesirable side effects. In contrast, acupuncture presents itself as an effective and side-effect-free alternative.

Acupuncture Outperforms Medication with No Side Effects

In a 2009 study published in the Journal of Clinical Oncology spanning 12 weeks, 47 breast cancer patients volunteered for either antidepressant (venlafaxine) treatment or acupuncture therapy. While the antidepressant group experienced diminished severity of hot flashes, they reported adverse effects such as anxiety, dizziness, fatigue, headaches, elevated blood pressure, nausea, and sleep disturbances.

Conversely, the acupuncture group witnessed a significant reduction in hot flashes without any observed side effects. Moreover, even after the cessation of therapy, hot flashes remained minimal for up to 15 weeks in the acupuncture group, contrasting with the resurgence of discomfort within two weeks of antidepressant cessation.

Acupuncture Alleviates Hot Flashes in Majority of Women

In September 2016, another study delved into this matter. The research encompassed 209 participants, all experiencing at least four hot flashes daily, either due to menopause or post-menopause. Half of the women underwent 20 acupuncture sessions over six months, while the remaining served as the control group without acupuncture.

The findings revealed:

- 11 percent of women who received acupuncture witnessed an 85 percent reduction in hot flashes after 8 weeks.

- 47 percent of women who underwent acupuncture reported a 47 percent decrease in hot flashes.

- 37 percent of women who received acupuncture experienced a nearly 10 percent reduction in hot flashes.
- In the control group, 80 percent experienced a modest 10 percent reduction in hot flashes.

This study underscores acupuncture's efficacy in mitigating hot flashes for the majority of menopausal women, making it a promising avenue for therapy worth exploring.

Acupuncture for Sleep Troubles

Addressing sleep disorders with acupuncture is best entrusted to a proficient practitioner. Traditional Chinese Medicine (TCM) attributes sleep disturbances to an energetic imbalance in the fire element, often stemming from Yin deficiency.

There exist more than 20 acupuncture points that can be targeted to address sleep issues. Typically, a few sessions under the guidance of an adept acupuncturist can effectively manage difficulties in falling asleep. However, for severe cases, around 20 or sometimes more sessions may be required.

Acupuncture for Reducing Dependency on Sleep Medications

Acupuncture can serve as a complementary approach to easing individuals off chemically synthesized sleep medications. Over several weeks, acupuncture is administered concurrently with a gradual reduction or tapering of the sleeping pill dosage.

By combining acupuncture with a gradual reduction of medication, the often unpleasant withdrawal symptoms associated with discontinuing sleep medication, such as restlessness or insomnia, can often be alleviated.

Upon completion of therapy, many individuals can discontinue sleep medication altogether, returning to natural, restorative sleep without the need for assistance.

Acupuncture for Osteoarthritis: A Traditional Approach

In the treatment of osteoarthritis, acupuncture, a cornerstone of traditional Chinese medicine, has stood the test of time. Its aim is to rebalance Qi and enhance blood circulation by stimulating specific points along the body's meridians.

By delicately inserting needles into these points, acupuncturists can alleviate Qi and blood blockages, thereby reducing the inflammation, stiffness, and pain characteristic of osteoarthritis. Moreover, acupuncture prompts the release of endorphins, the body's natural pain-relievers, further diminishing discomfort.

Acupuncture Points Tailored for Osteoarthritis

Numerous acupuncture points are applicable in addressing osteoarthritis, with the selection depending on the location of pain and the patient's specific symptoms.

For instance, in knee osteoarthritis cases, points like "Stomach 36" (E36) on the leg and "Bladder 60" (V60) at the ankle's rear may be utilized. E36 is often chosen for its Qi and blood strengthening properties, along with its inflammation and pain-alleviating effects, while V60 is renowned for its efficacy in lower body pain relief.

The Procedure of Osteoarthritis Treatment through Acupuncture

In an acupuncture session targeting osteoarthritis, practitioners typically commence with a comprehensive consultation, delving into pain characteristics, medical history, lifestyle, and dietary habits. This aids in identifying underlying energy imbalances contributing to osteoarthritis.

Subsequently, specific acupuncture points are selected and stimulated to rectify Qi and blood balance. Needles remain in place for 20 to 30 minutes, during which patients may experience sensations like warmth, tingling, or heaviness around the needle insertion sites.

Acupuncture as a Component of Holistic Osteoarthritis Management

It is vital to recognize that acupuncture is often incorporated alongside other osteoarthritis treatments. Lifestyle adjustments, including a nutritious diet and regular exercise, can significantly reduce inflammation and manage pain.

Moreover, complementary traditional Chinese medicine therapies like Tui Na (a form of Chinese massage) may enhance acupuncture's efficacy when used concurrently. Ultimately, the objective is to devise a holistic treatment regimen addressing not just the physical manifestations of osteoarthritis, but also the underlying energetic imbalances contributing to the ailment.

Relieving Nausea and Vomiting with Acupressure

Acupressure, derived from Chinese medicine and akin to acupuncture, offers relief by stimulating specific points on the body.

To alleviate nausea and vomiting, focus on a point near the wrist.

To practice acupressure, apply pressure using your thumb, index finger, or middle finger. Position your fingertip at the center of the point and massage in a clockwise direction. Your finger should make 2 or 3 circles per second. Maintain contact with the skin but avoid using the nail to press.

This acupressure technique can be applied for 5 minutes prior to chemotherapy and before meals. It can also be performed at the onset of nausea.

Alternatively, wearing an acupressure bracelet can provide similar benefits to manual massage.

Position the ring finger along the wrist's flexion crease, with the desired

point corresponding to the height of
the index finger.

Acupuncture in Pregnancy Care

An increasing number of obstetricians are integrating acupuncture into their care for pregnant women, either as an alternative or complement to conventional medical practices. This ancient therapy has gained recognition within midwifery.

Many expectant mothers seek alternative treatments to address pregnancy-related symptoms or prepare for childbirth, finding acupuncture to be an effective option.

Acupuncture for Pregnancy Symptoms

The journey of pregnancy is accompanied by a range of physical and emotional changes, and acupuncture offers relief for various issues:

Sleep disturbances: Acupuncture sessions, typically administered an hour before bedtime, can often alleviate sleep troubles.

Morning sickness: Acupuncture may offer relief for more severe cases of morning sickness, beyond the effectiveness of common home remedies.

Heartburn: Regular acupuncture targeting specific points can reduce the incidence of heartburn, a common discomfort in later stages of pregnancy.

Sciatica and back pain: By stimulating specific acupuncture points, these common pregnancy complaints can be eased.

Headaches and migraines: Acupuncture is known to effectively manage headaches, a benefit that extends to pregnancy-related discomfort.

Carpal tunnel syndrome: Symptoms like wrist numbness and pain, often exacerbated during pregnancy, may find relief through acupuncture.

Initial improvements from acupuncture therapy are typically noticeable after three to six sessions, with chronic issues requiring additional time for symptom alleviation.

Acupuncture for Birth Preparation

Acupuncture's efficacy in pain management makes it a popular choice for birth preparation, with sessions commonly sought before and during labor.

Prenatal Acupuncture

Expectant mothers, especially those opting for natural childbirth, often explore methods to manage labor pain. Prenatal acupuncture aims to promote relaxation and reduce pre-birth anxieties, potentially shortening labor duration and reducing the need for pain medication.

Starting from the 36th week of pregnancy, weekly acupuncture sessions may be recommended until delivery to support cervical maturation and facilitate smoother labor progression.

While childbirth timing remains unpredictable, acupuncture can be utilized to stimulate labor when the body is deemed ready for delivery, potentially easing the waiting period post due date.

Acupuncture During Childbirth

Acupuncture can offer significant assistance not only throughout pregnancy but also during childbirth by alleviating pain. It often induces relaxation and provides pain relief akin to analgesics, minus the potential side effects.

However, acupuncture should be viewed as a complementary method and should not replace established obstetric interventions. The specific placement of needles during labor acupuncture varies depending on individual circumstances and should be administered by a skilled practitioner.

In place of needle acupuncture, manual stimulation of acupuncture points, known as acupressure, can serve as an alternative during labor as well as pregnancy.

How Acupuncture Treatment Typically Operates

Both physicians and midwives can undergo additional training to become acupuncture therapists. Consult with your midwife and/or obstetrician to determine when acupuncture might be recommended to prepare for childbirth and how to locate a qualified practitioner.

Every acupuncture session should begin with a comprehensive health assessment, particularly crucial during pregnancy.

During your initial consultation with an acupuncturist, gather detailed information about the treatment approach to determine its suitability for you.

A typical session lasts around 20 minutes, during which you'll likely be in a comfortable position. If acupuncture is incorporated during labor, mobility is limited, making it convenient to have the needles inserted during routine CTG monitoring, where movement is restricted anyway.

Potential Risks of Acupuncture During Pregnancy

Acupuncture, whether administered during labor or as a prenatal measure, carries some risks:

Minor skin injuries like bleeding

Risk of infections

Potential side effects such as dizziness, nausea, low blood pressure, and fatigue

Bruising at needle insertion points

Difficulty in removing forgotten needles

While complications are rare, it's essential to be aware of them before starting acupuncture treatment during pregnancy. Generally, acupuncture sessions are painless and free from complications.

Since there's limited research on the effects of acupuncture during pregnancy and childbirth, it's not covered by statutory health insurance. Therefore, the costs of acupuncture are typically paid out of pocket by the pregnant woman. However, some health insurance plans may partially cover acupuncture for specific pregnancy-related issues, so it's advisable to inquire about coverage options.

Key Points to Consider

When is acupuncture useful during pregnancy?

Acupuncture can help alleviate early pregnancy symptoms like headaches or nausea. Prenatal acupuncture is typically initiated around the 36th week of pregnancy.

What are the potential benefits of acupuncture during pregnancy?

Acupuncture has a wide range of applications during pregnancy, from treating pregnancy symptoms and reducing anxiety to providing pain relief and promoting relaxation during childbirth.

How frequently can acupuncture sessions be scheduled during pregnancy?

The frequency of acupuncture treatments required before

experiencing initial results varies depending on the specific condition. Therefore, detailed consultation is necessary before starting therapy.

Can acupuncture harm the baby during pregnancy?

There are no known adverse effects on the unborn baby associated with acupuncture. Increased fetal movements might occur after a session.

Moreover, even during the postnatal period, acupuncture may offer relief from certain postnatal symptoms while aiding in the recovery phase after childbirth.

Acupuncture as a Strategy for Weight Management

Acupuncture is increasingly utilized as a method for weight loss, targeting appetite and weight regulation. Its efficacy lies in addressing various factors that disrupt inner balance, leading to appetite disorders and weight gain:

1. Stress
2. Anxiety
3. Hormonal imbalance

By addressing these factors, acupuncture aids in weight loss by promoting healthy eating habits aligned with genuine hunger cues, thus facilitating weight reduction and achieving desired weight goals.

How Acupuncture Facilitates Weight Loss

1. Appetite Control: Acupuncture assists in controlling appetite, enabling individuals to adjust their hunger levels and modify eating behaviors to consume only what is necessary for their nutritional needs, thereby facilitating weight loss.

2. Regulation of Hunger Hormone: Acupuncture regulates ghrelin levels, often referred to as the "hunger hormone," which influences the desire to snack between meals, contributing to better appetite management and weight loss.

3. Mitigation of Emotional Eating: Emotional eating, characterized by eating in response to emotional stress, is countered by acupuncture through stress reduction, thereby curbing cravings for fatty or sugary foods triggered by negative emotions.

Procedure of Acupuncture Sessions for Weight Loss

During an acupuncture session, the practitioner strategically places fine needles on specific points of the patient's body. The patient lies down and is encouraged to relax while the practitioner applies the needles to targeted energy points. The process is painless as the needles are extremely thin and only penetrate the surface of the skin.

Energy points vary for each individual based on their unique body composition, health status, lifestyle, and experiences. Typically lasting an hour, an acupuncture session may involve multiple sessions scheduled weekly over a period of 2 to 4 months to observe significant weight loss results. However, the number and duration of sessions may vary depending on individual circumstances.

It's important to understand that acupuncture alone is not a magic solution for weight loss. It can yield genuine results when incorporated into a comprehensive weight loss program. Adopting a balanced diet and engaging in regular physical activity are essential components for shedding pounds in a healthy and sustainable manner. Acupuncture addresses symptoms such as appetite by rebalancing the body's energy flows but does not directly tackle the root cause of overweight.

Furthermore, it's crucial to distinguish acupuncture from auriculotherapy, a similar method used for weight loss. Unlike acupuncture, auriculotherapy involves placing a single staple on specific points of the ear's cartilage, rather than needles on various points of the body. While the methods differ, both aim to regulate appetite and facilitate weight loss.

Chapter 11

**Frequently Asked Questions
Faq: Common Queries Regarding
Acupuncture**

Does acupuncture work effectively?

Acupuncture's effectiveness has been backed by numerous scientific studies. The World Health Organization (WHO) in 2003 listed 28 conditions where acupuncture surpasses placebo effectiveness. Over 13,000 studies conducted across 60 nations since then have demonstrated its efficacy in treating 117 syndromes.

Is needle insertion painful?

Acupuncture needles are remarkably thin and cause minimal discomfort. They are sterile and approximately 20 times thinner than those used for drawing blood, akin to the width of a hair. Sensations during acupuncture are often likened to a mosquito bite, with a dull or electric shock-like feeling. Even individuals with needle phobia can undergo acupuncture treatment without issue, as needles are single-use.

What attire should I wear for acupuncture sessions?

Comfortable clothing and underwear are recommended. Alternatively, we provide shorts and a t-shirt or camisole if preferred. During the treatment, you will be draped with a paper sheet for privacy.

How many sessions are needed to address my condition?

The number of treatments required varies depending on the severity, chronicity, age, and health status of the condition. Typically, 3 to 6 sessions are needed to achieve significant improvement in an imbalance.

What is the duration of an acupuncture session?
The initial consultation typically lasts about 1 hour and 15 minutes. Subsequent sessions range from 45 to 60 minutes.

Is belief in acupuncture necessary for its effectiveness?
No, a positive bias towards acupuncture is not a prerequisite for its efficacy. It can effectively treat individuals, including children,

without any preconceived notions about the practice.

Can my condition worsen after acupuncture?

Acupuncture generally does not have adverse effects. However, in rare instances, it may trigger a mild inflammatory reaction due to the body's natural healing mechanisms, lasting up to 24 to 48 hours. Following this reaction, symptoms typically decrease significantly.

Chinese medicine versus conventional medicine?

Chinese medicine is typically sought when conventional medicine fails to resolve issues. It is particularly effective for functional disorders, while conventional medicine is better suited for organic or biological problems, such as bacterial infections treated with antibiotics rather than acupuncture.